Whole Foods Plant-Based Lifestyle Guidebook

Written

By

Catherine Grace Fleming

Copyright © 2021 by Catherine Fleming
Whole Foods Plant-Based Lifestyle Guidebook
(BKR853-C5) ISBN: 978-1-7372220-0-2

First Edition.

All rights reserved. No part of this book may be reproduced in any manner whatsoever without written permission except in the case of brief quotations embodied in critical articles and reviews.

First Printing, 2021

This is dedicated to those concerned about the health and well being in ourselves, society, Mother Earth, and all living beings.

And to my children whom I love with all my heart. I hope to help create a sustainable planet for them to live a long healthy life.
- C.G.F.

I'm one of those people that likes things that are straightforward and easy to follow. I want to dive in but not read 100's of pages beforehand. I want to take action right away. I hope I have made this guidebook just that.

~The Basics~

Eat complex carbs, no oil, a low amount of whole food fats, and a small amount or no sugar.

What are complex carbs? Vegetables, fruits, beans, potatoes, and whole grains.

Fats: Avocado, tahini, nuts and seeds, and nut butters.

Fiber: Beans, Whole Grains (Rice, Quinoa, Oats,etc), fruits, and a Rainbow of Vegetables.

Add sparkle: herbs and spices, aminos, miso, and oil free condiments

Sugars: Small amounts of maple syrup, or maple sugar, and substitutes like date paste (date paste can be used in almost any recipe), stevia leaf, not the powder (stay away from anything that is white and powdery).

Supplements, Necessary to Live A Healthy Life

- B12 (Premier Research Labs is my fave) - a few times/week, check your levels to see what you need. See videos about B12 at *nutritonfacts.org* and why EVERYONE needs them, even meat eaters.

- D3 (Premier Research Labs, again my fave) - depending on what your blood panel tells you. A guideline is 4 drops for adults, 2 drops for kids.

- DHA/Omega 3's: ground flax, hemp, walnuts, chia are all good sources.
    - I use walnuts on my oats in the morning and ground flax on my salads. Chia can also be put in oats, in Nice Cream, frosting, etc. More on DHA and Omega 3's at *nutrtionfacts.org*

- Iodine: seaweed or supplement. I just add seaweed to my salad dressing. Check your levels as low iodine can affect your thyroid.

- Sauerkraut or Other Fermented Foods
    - Feeds the bacteria in your gut like a probiotic.
    - Ex. Sauerkraut, kimchi, pickles
    - Brands I recommend
        - Bubbies©
        - So many new companies making fermented foods, try each one until you find what you like
        - Make your own - *Simnett Nutrition* on YouTube has a great tutorial
    - **Not** canned pickles or sauerkraut - good bacteria is killed in the canning process

Condiments

- Mustard
    - Yellow, brown, spicy, etc.
- Primal Kitchen© Ketchup, Barbecue sauce, etc.
- Sauce recipe (see recipe section)
- Make your own sauces and salsas from cook books in the reference section.
- Salsa - can be put on almost anything
- Tamari (Braggs is our favorite)
- Hummus (look for brands with NO OIL)
    - Recipes in Esselstyn books

Cookware

- Glass, stainless steel, cast iron, and silicone are best
- Plastic leaches into your food
- Non-stick cookware can off-gas toxic fumes and is environmentally toxic (watch *Dark Waters* with Mark Ruffalo and Anne Hathaway).
- Aluminum can leach into your food as well as you cook.

Set Yourself Up for Success

- Clean out your kitchen
- Kitchen essentials for success
    - 2 pots with lids
    - Steaming pot and insert
    - Baking dish
    - Thrift stores are stocked with many of these items
- Swap out simple and processed carbohydrates for complex carbohydrates
- Make substitutions of your favorite processed foods
- Bring snacks and meals with you
- Keep it simple
    - Make big batches of the staples
        - Rice, beans, potatoes, steamed veg, etc.
    - Use convenience foods when necessary
        - Canned beans (no oil or extra salt)
        - Frozen vegetables
        - Hummus (no oil or tahini)
        - Salsa

- Buy an Instapot
    - A larger size can leave you with leftovers for days
- Do it on the cheap
    - Buy in bulk
        - Rice, beans, nuts, seeds, etc.
        - Order bulk from your local natural food store or grocery chain.
    - Make your own
        - Tahini (ground sesame seeds in a food processor)
        - Date paste (food processor with a little water)
        - Almond butter (food processor)
- Baby food grinder
    - Anything you eat baby can too
    - Manual grinder to take anywhere
    - Power hand blender for home
- **Be kind to yourself. If you eat junk, pick yourself up, dust off and do better next time. It *is* a process, even for those with the best intentions. Focus on the fact that most of the time you are eating well.**

Beans and Legumes
- Pinto, garbanzo, kidney, black, your favorite
- Buy canned if more convenient for your lifestyle
  - Look for beans with NO OIL
- Bean pasta is good mixed with rice pasta

Lentils
- Any color is fine
- Soak with apple cider vinegar, 24 hours
- Rinse and cook

Soy beans
- Can help regulate your hormones - see Dr. Neal Barnard's Book *Your Body in Balance*
- ½ cup a day
- Cook like beans
- Tofu - can scramble like eggs or cube and add to rice and veg, etc.
  - We find it best to marinade, lots of recipes in the books section or Simnett Nutrition YouTube videos

Cooking/Sprouting Beans and Legumes
- Instapot - easiest and fastest way to cook beans, rice and potatoes
- Sprouting - for 3 days in jars - can be eaten that way - refer to Doug Evans *Sprouts* book

Whole Grains and Tubers

- Quinoa - rinse well before cooking
- Rice - basmati or jasmine (white or brown fine). Rice Pasta is ok too.
    - Soak overnight with apple cider vinegar OR rinse 4 times before cooking
    - Cook with a ¼ cup less water - depending how dry or sticky you want it
- Oats - soak overnight or 8 hours with apple cider vinegar - easier to digest
    - Oat flour can be used in many recipes instead of wheat
    - Starting with oats for breakfast is ideal
- Sweet potato, yam or potato - serve any way you like
    - Hummus or salsa on top is great
    - Cook at 400° for 1 hour, steam, or mash
- Whole Wheat
    - Can be hard on the gut. Be mindful of what your body tells you when you eat wheat
    - Recommended brand
        - Ezekiel Brand

Steamed Vegetables
- 3 - 6 cups a day
- Eat your Rainbow every day for overall health
    - Rutabagas - 1/2 inch cubes and/or Beets
    - Cabbage (red or chinese)
    - Broccoli, Brussel Sprouts, or Asparagus
    - Cauliflower (add in colored cauli when avail.)
    - White, red, and yellow onion
    - Greens
        - Kale, swiss chard, beet greens, mustard, etc.
    - Garlic
    - Mushroom

Steam enough for 2-3 days at a time. For convenience steam on Sunday and Wednesday. My steamer takes 14-16 minutes, yours may take longer or shorter time, check often the first few times by poking the beets or rutabagas, if they skewer through easily they are done. More notes on steaming veg under recipes. **Save the steaming water and use in soups, stews and/or for making refried beans.**

Salad
- Lettuce, bok choy, massaged kale, and/or chinese cabbage
- Raw mushroom - 1 to 2 or more slices
- Sunflower seeds - sprinkle on - dry roasted is fine, no oil
- Tomato, cucumber, bell pepper, etc
- Fruit (optional) apples, grapes, or pear are nice
- Sauerkraut/kimchi or other fermented foods, not canned
- Additions:
    - Nutritional yeast
    - Lemon
    - Balsamic vinegar
    - Sea salt
    - Sauce - in recipe section
    - Turmeric
    - Black pepper
    - Cayenne

Fruits
- Berries - all kinds, especially wild blueberries
- Bananas, apples, and goji berries are staples
- Any other fruits - we love mangoes
- Dates for smoothies and as a sweetener

Fats

- Avocado
- Tahini
- Nut butters (except peanut butter, all have mold spores) almond preferable
- Nuts (brazil, walnut, almond)
- Seeds (sunflower seeds, pumpkin) no oil
- Stay away from oils
- If you need to gain weight - eat a little more from this section
- If you need to lose weight - eat less from this section

Other Foods To Add

- Chia seeds (blended in smoothie, on your cereal, salad, beans, and/or grains)
- Maca powder - helps with energy in afternoon (blended in smoothie)
- Miso (add to soup, sauce and grain and bean dishes)
- Aminos (Braggs brand or organic low sodium type)
- Spices and Herbs

The Plate Method

½ Plate
Salad & Steamed Veg
¼ Plate
Whole grain or Potato
¼ Plate Beans, lentils or tofu

(Pictures at SpreadingWellness.org)

What I Eat in a Day
Sample of a Simple Meal Day

Guideline: ½ of your plate is salad and steamed vegetables. ¼ is a whole grain or potato. ¼ is a type of legume.

Breakfast
- Oatmeal with Blueberries, walnuts, and hemp on top
- Salad with steam veg and small amount of soy or refried beans on top (optional, but so good - mood booster, see Neal Barnard's book *Your Body in Balance*)

Snack: fruit

Lunch
- Salad with steam veg on top or side
  - Salad Dressing
  - Beans added to salad if not in meal
- Refried beans and rice with salsa and avocado with or without tortilla (organic sprouted corn or Ezekiel's Sprouted Wheat)
- Or Sweet potato/potato with beans

Snack
- Fruit, Smoothie, nIce Cream, popcorn (no oil, braggs spray is nice with some nutritional yeast)

Dinner
- Same as lunch

Keep it simple and expand later. You will find what you like and have extra on hand for easy meals.

Remember
This is a lifestyle, not a diet. This is a way of eating you can sustain for the rest of your life.
How Much to Eat (Most folks don't know that you need to eat more when eating this way). These sites can help.
https://plantspace.org/caloric-needs-calculator/ and *https://cronometer.com/*

~Recipes~

Oats
- 2 c. Oat Groats
- Cover with water by ½"
- 1T of Apple Cider Vinegar
- Soak overnight or 8 hours
- Rinse
- Blend in a blender or food processor until they look like steel cut oats
- Place in a pot
- Add 2 cups water for every cup of oats
- Sea Salt - ½ t for every 2 cups of oats

Directions: Put your oats on medium heat until they start to simmer. Turn down to low and cook for 30-45 minutes until done. Scrape off the bottom of the pot every 5 to 10 minutes. I have found that using oat groats are so much sweeter and easier to digest. My kids put less sugar on these because they don't need it. I add Cinnamon, blueberries, walnuts, hemp seeds, and sometimes a banana. Supplements that can be added are chlorella and mushroom powder for example.

My kids add maple syrup and homemade carob chips.

Recipes for all kinds of oats in the Esselstyn's books and YouTube videos. (See resources)

Cathy's Pancakes
- 1 T ground flax
- 3 T water
- 1 t of almond butter
- 1 -2 pinches sea salt
- 1/2 t baking soda
- 1/2 t vanilla
- Oats - cooked
- Buckwheat groat flour (can ground groats yourself)
- Water
- Blueberries (frozen or fresh)

Directions: Soak the ground flax in the 3 T water for 10 minutes (this is a flax egg). After 10 minutes add the almond butter and whisk in. Mix in the salt, baking soda, and vanilla. Whisk in enough cooked oats to your liking or until consistency is almost too thick. Start adding flour(s) and water until it's thick and goopy or thinner to your liking. Fold in blueberries. Heat up the pan or griddle for 5 minutes before pouring on batter. Since I don't use any oil in my kitchen I use a stainless steel spatula that scrapes the pancakes off the pan easily. Heat up the pan for 5 minutes before pouring on batter. Makes about 6 pancakes. Double or triple this recipe if needed.

Cinnamon Oatmeal Breakfast (or anytime) Cookies

(modified from *Simnett Nutrition's Recipe* from YouTube *"Oats are Amazing & Why You Should Eat Them"*)

- 2 bananas
- Smash
- ½ cup of almond butter
- ¼ t sea salt
- 1 to 2 t cinnamon
- Mix in
- 1 ½ cups of rolled oats
- Mix in
- ¼ to ½ cup raisins, chocolate chips, or carob chips
- Fold in

Directions: Put about 1 ½ to 2 T of cookie batter on a cookie sheet for 15 - 17 minutes at 350 degrees.

Steamed Veg

- I steam root veg, cabbage, cauliflower, brussel sprouts, broccoli, and onion for 9 minutes.
- After 9 minutes I add mushrooms, greens, garlic, and any frozen veg and steam for another 6 minutes.
- I then check the root veg. If my fork or knife can easily go through, it is ready, if not, cook for 2 more minutes and check again.
- We want to be able to put a knife into the veg easily and the veg be brightly colored, but not limp and slimy.
- Each color you eat symbolizes a body system - eat the rainbow for your whole body health.

Note: Save steaming water for soup or in lieu of water for rice or quinoa (lots of vitamins and minerals in that water) - huge to help heal the body

Pasta

- We eat pasta once or twice a week. The whole grain or bean equivalent is best.
- Marinara or dairy and oil free pesto is good on top.

Cooking Beans
- Soak overnight to 24 hours with 2T of apple cider vinegar per 4 cups of beans
    - Rinse
    - cook for 4 hours or less
    - easier to digest if you soak first, otherwise you might be "tooting" more
- Soak 12 cups at a time, freeze in Pint or quart jars for the month.

Refried Beans - My Version

- Pint to a quart of cooked beans (I use black, kidney, and pinto mix)
- Add steamed veg water - when it peeks out from under beans is enough
- 1-2 T of miso
- ½ to 1 t or less of sea salt
- 1 T or more of Chili Powder or other spice (Ex. Curry, Taco Seasoning)
- 1 clove or more of garlic
- Pepper to taste

Directions: Put all ingredients in a pot on Medium. Let bubble and cook as you stir every once in a while, smashing with the back of a wooden or stainless steel spoon or with a potato masher. Cook down and turn down heat as you go and scrape the beans off the bottom of the pan until almost all the liquid has evaporated. Serve with rice or potato, with or without a wrap. Yum!

Smoothie Base - Good as is
- 1 banana
- Berries - handful
- Kale - 1 leaf
- 1 - 2 dates (optional)
- Oat milk (organic) or water - pour in a little at a time to your liking

Additions - add nutrition to your smoothie - can be very tasty
- 1 T Goji berries
- 1-2 T Hemp seed
- 1 T Almond butter or more
- 2 t chia seed
- 3 brazil nuts - good selenium source
- ½ pinch of sea salt
    - Additions
        - Maca (for an energy boost)
        - Cinnamon
        - Spirulina
        - Ginger
- Double or triple if sharing

Sauce or Salad Dressing - for salads and beans and rice or potato
(Adapted from *Simnett Nutrition*'s Sauce Recipes on YouTube)
- ⅓ cup of Tahini
- 1 - 2 T Miso
- 1-3 t of Ground Flax
- 1-2 t of Nutritional Yeast
- 2 t Apple cider vinegar
- 1 - 2 T Balsamic vinegar or more
- 1-2 t of Date Paste
- 2 t Seaweed - dulse, kelp, nori or your fave (Mountain Rose herbs .com)
- Pepper to taste (optional)
- Turmeric - couple shakes (optional)
- Water - to your preferred consistency
- Variations : mustard instead of balsamic vinegar

Directions: Put all ingredients in a bowl, add water a little at a time and whisk in until it's a consistency of your liking. Taste, add more date paste or balsamic vinegar to your liking. Scrape with spatula to make sure all tahini is mixed in. Put in the fridge. Lasts 5 days.

Dirty Rice
- Saute ¼ onion, 1 to 2 stalks of celery with ¼ cup of Veg broth added a little at a time while sauteing
- Saute ~ 3 minutes
- Cooked Rice - add 2 cups or more
- Amino acids or Tamari
- Pepper and sea salt to your liking
- 1-2 t of Ginger root slice in garlic press, add during last 2 minutes of cooking with lid on

My husband and son love dirty rice!

Soup Base
- Veg stock - liquid from steamed veg
- Miso 1-2 t or more depending on how much liquid you have
- Sea salt to taste
- Pepper - few shakes
- Aminos (optional)
- We drink this in mugs once a day just as is because it is so good for you (lots of vitamins and minerals).
- Or I saute onion, mushroom and celery first and then add everything, but I also use this as the liquid for my rice or to refried beans.

Oat Seed Bread

(modified from an original recipe by Eve Supica)

- 3 cups Oats (rolled or steel cut)
- 2 cups Sunflower seeds
- 1 cup Flax seeds
- 1 cup Pumpkin seeds
- ½ cup Ground Flax seed (to bind bread together)
- ¼ cup Chia seeds
- 2 t Salt
- 2 T Date paste
- 6 T Tahini
- 3 cups water

Directions: Mix all ingredients together and pour into 2 loaf pans (silicone pans work really well with this recipe). Let rest for a few hours or overnight to absorb liquid.
Bake in loaf pans for 30 min. At 350°. Remove from pans and place the half-cooked loaves on a cookie sheet. Bake for another 30 minutes at 350°. Cool before slicing. Keep in Fridge.

Oat Seed Bread Variations:
- Crackers - spread on 2 cookie sheets - silicone or on parchment paper. Bake at 350° for 30min, flip and 30 min more.
- Pizza - use 1/3rd of the recipe for each pizza crust. Spread out on a pizza sheet or stone and bake 20 to 30 minutes at 350°, flip and another 20-30 minutes on the other side. Can be picked up and eaten.

Mom's Guacamole

- 1 Avocado
- ⅛ thin slice of onion
- 1 to 2 small spoonfuls salsa
- Salt and pepper to taste
- lemon juice to taste

Directions: Blend together until smooth in a food processor or blender. Eat right away or chill for 30 minutes and serve.

Flax Egg
- 1 T of ground flax
- 3 T of water
- Substitutes one egg

How to Saute
- Add water or Veg broth when sauteing.

Eating Out
- *Happy Cow* website - find a place to eat almost anywhere
- Order steam vegetables and rice
- Salad without dressing, add vinegar or lemon on the side with beans
- *My Beef with Meat* by Rip Esselstyn has some great tips in his book.

Athletes

After starting on a Whole Foods Plant-Based (WFPB) Lifestyle of eating you will notice more energy. I have read and heard more stories than I can count of folks becoming athletic after going WFPB. The cells are no longer covered in fat and the energy flow is uninhibited into your muscles and cells (see Mastering Diabetes in resources). Here are some tips and supplements to help increase your ability to maximize your body's performance and repair. (See *Simnett Nutrition's* YouTube channel for more info).

- Cordyceps Mushrooms - may increase lung capacity
    - Add to smoothies or cereal
    - Host Defense© Mushrooms or Mountain Rose Herbs© has them
- Beet juicing/crystals - may increase blood flow to muscles
    - Add to green juice or water
    - Drink first thing in am or before a workout
- Hawthorn or Blueberries
    - Can increase circulation
    - Can decrease inflammation
    - Can protects Heart and Capillaries for sustained performance
- Celery Juice
    - Can give a good pump when working out
    - Detoxes and energizes

Grocery List - Try your best to eat as much organic as you can

Veg
- Lettuce
- Tomato, cucumber, bell pepper, etc for salad
- Avocado
- White, red, and yellow onion
- Cauliflower (add in colored cauli when avail.)
- Beets
- Broccoli
- Greens 1-2 bunches for steamed and smoothies
    - Kale, swiss chard, beet greens, mustard, any will do
- Cabbage (red or chinese)
- Rutabagas
- Garlic
- Mushroom
- Celery
- Sweet Potato/Yam
- Potatoes
- Lemons
- Ginger root

Fruit
- Bananas
- Berries - blueberries, strawberries, blackberries, raspberries
- Apple
- Goji berries
- Dates
- Raisins - (no added oil)
- Any other fruits you like

Nuts/Seeds
- Almonds
- Almond butter
- Brazil nuts
- Roasted Sunflower Seeds (No oil)
- Walnuts
- Pumpkin Seeds
- Chia Seeds
- Hemp Seeds
- Flax seeds (ground or whole)
- Any other nuts or seeds you like

Beans/Legumes
- Pinto, black, garbanzo, and/or kidney
- Lentils - any color
- Soy beans
- Tofu (optional)

Grains
- Rice - Basmati or Jasmine (brown)
- Quinoa
- Oats - groats and rolled
- Ezekial Bread
- Popcorn
- Buckwheat groats or flour

Miscellaneous:
- Miso
- Tamari (low salt) or Amino Acids
- Apple Cider Vinegar
- Tahini or sesame seeds to make own
- Sauerkraut - raw (Bubbies or other brand) or other raw ferments (kimchi)
- Balsamic vinegar
- Oat milk or Soy milk
- Seaweed - dulse or nori (*https://www.mountainroseherbs.com/*)
- Sprouted corn or Ezekiel tortillas
- Maca (good for energy boost)
- Vanilla
- Maple syrup
- Chocolate Chips
- Beet Juice Crystals
- Salsa
- Baking Soda

Spices
- Sea salt
- Turmeric
- Black pepper
- Cayenne (optional, but good for digestion)
- Chili Powder
- Nutritional yeast
- Cinnamon - ceylon is best
- Spices and Herbs of choice

Research and Resources

Start here
- *Mastering Diabetes* by Dr. Cyrus Khambatta and Robby Barbaro (whether your diabetic or not, they will teach you the importance of insulin sensitivity)
- *Your Body in Balance* by Neal Barnard
- *Fiber Fueled* by Will Bulsiewicz
- *Prevent and Reverse Heart Disease* by Dr. Caldwell Esselstyn
- *www.pcrm.org* Look up: *Vegan Diet Better for Weight Loss and Cholesterol Control than Mediterranean Diet*
- *72 Reasons to be Vegan* by Gene Stone and Kathy Freston

For more research
- Dr. T. Colin Campbell
  - *The China Study*
  - *Whole*
  - *The Future of Nutrition*
- Dr. Michael Gregor
  - *How Not To Die*
  - *How Not To Die Cookbook*
  - *How Not to Diet*
  - *How to Survive a Pandemic*
- Dr. Neal Barnard
  - *The Cheese Trap*
- *The Pleasure Trap* by Alan Goldhamer and Dr. Douglas J. Lisle

- *The Starch Solution* by John McDougal
- *Breasts: The Owner's Manual* by Kristi Funk

Research Websites
- *NutritionFacts.org*
- *NutritionStudies.org*

Recipe Books
- *The Prevent and Reverse Heart Disease Cookbook* by Anne and Jane Esselstyn
- *The Engine 2 Cookbook* by Rip and Jane Esselstyn
- *The Sprout Book* by Doug Evans
- *My Beef With Meat* by Rip Esselstyn
- *The Healthiest Diet on the Planet* by Dr. John McDougall and Mary McDougall

YouTubers and Podcasts
- *Simnett Nutrition* on YouTube
- *Jane Esselstyn* on YouTube - super fun videos with her mom
- *Rich Roll* YouTube and Podcast
- *Switch 4 Good* YouTube and Podcast
- *Mic The Vegan* on YouTube
- *PlantStrong* by Rip Esselstyn YouTube and Podcast
- *Chef AJ* on YouTube
- *Physicians Committee* on YouTube

YouTubers and Podcasts cont.
- *Plant Based Science London* on YouTube
- *NutritonFacts.org* on YouTube
- *TheRawAdvantage* YouTube
- *Earthling Ed* YouTube
- *The Real Truth About Health* YouTube
- *Alan Goldhamer* YouTube
- *Veg Source* YouTube
- *Mastering Diabetes* YouTube

Movies
- *Gamechangers* (Netflix)
- *Forks Over Knives*
- *The Invisible Vegan* (AmazonPrime)
- *Cowspiracy* (Netflix)
- *What the Health* (Netflix)
- *Vegan Stories*
- *Earthlings* (Narrated by Joaquin Phoenix, Netflix)
- *Seaspiracy* (Netflix)

Note: Also look for these books and videos at your local library.

Books About Animal Rights
- *https://www.peta.org/living/entertainment/animal-rights-books/*

Books and Products to Look Into After You Get the Basics Down

- Herbs
    - *Herbal Recipes for Vibrant Health* by Rosemary Gladstar
    - *Fire Cider: 101 Zesty Recipes* by Rosemary Gladstar
    - *Herbal Tonic Therapies* by Daniel Mowry, PhD
    - *Black Forager* on Instagram
    - *LearningHerbs.com*
- Mushrooms
    - *Medicinal Mushrooms* by Christopher Hobbs
    - Host Defense© Mushrooms
    - Stamets 7 powder is what we use.
        - Add to smoothies, sprinkle on or mix in cereal
    - Adds nutrients to your food and supports a healthy body

Index

Additions 13
Athletes 29
B12 3
Beans 8-9, 21-22
Cinnamon Oatmeal
Breakfast Cookies 19
Cathy's Pancakes 18
Condiments 5
Cookies 19
Cookware 5
Cronometer 15
D3 3
DHA 3
Dirty Rice 25
Eating Out 28
Fats 13
Fermented Foods 4
Flax Egg 28
Fruit 12
Grocery List 30-33
Guacamole 27
Herbs 37
How Much to Eat
Websites 15
Iodine 3
Lentils 8
Mom's Guacamole 27

Mushrooms 37
Oats 10, 17
Oat Seed Bread 26-27
Omega - 3's 3
Pancakes 18
Pasta 20
PlantSpace.org 15
The Plate Method 14-15
Potato 10
Recipes 17
Refried Beans 22
Salad 12
Salad Dressing 24
Sauce 24
Sauerkraut 4
Saute 28
Set Yourself Up For
Success 6-7
Smoothie 23
Soup Base 25
Soy Beans 8
Steamed Veg 11, 20
Supplements 3-4
Sweet Potatoes 10
Tubers 10
Whole Grains 10
Whole Wheat 10

Thank you!!

~Thanks to my husband for inspiring, nudging, and supporting me on this adventure. I really appreciate it. I love that you believe in me.

~Thank you to my sister, Sandra, who has always been there for me. I love you! Thank you for your continued support, editing and suggestions.

~Thank you also to my son, James, for helping with computer programs, converting files, and the book cover that you see. You have become invaluable to this modern world of electronics. I look forward to seeing where that takes you. I love you!

About the Author:

Cathy lives in the Northwoods of Wisconsin with her husband, 3 kids, 2 dogs, 2 cats, and 2 birds. She is a certified nutrition coach, lifetime herbology student, and lover of everything active. Often you can find her in the kitchen cooking food with her family, making some herbal concoction, in the garden or on her bike. Whole foods as her fuel.

Connect with Cathy

Instagram: cathy.spreading.wellness
YouTube: Cathy Spreading Wellness
Website: SpreadingWellness.org
Email: cathyspreadingwellness@gmail.com

Be kind to others,
take care of yourself so that you can be helpful
and kind to others,
exercise regularly (do something you love),
and meditate for 10 minutes a day.
~Namaste~

www.ingramcontent.com/pod-product-compliance
Lightning Source LLC
Chambersburg PA
CBHW020037120526
44589CB00032B/611